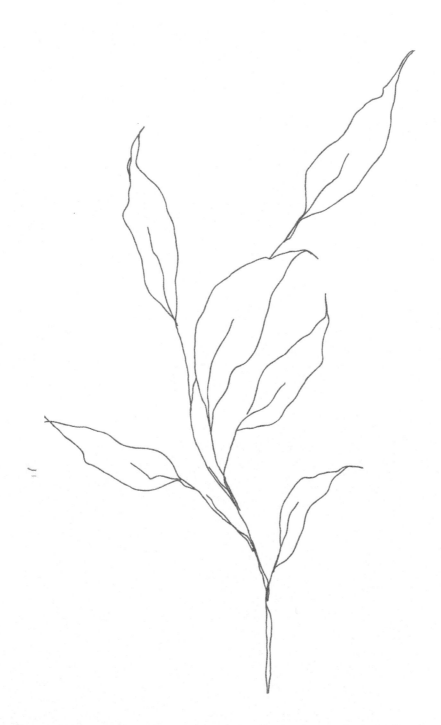

A Prayer for Your Health
JOURNAL

Reset, Reconnect, and Realign

This journal is a companion to the
Daniel Fast: A Bridge to Healthy Living
4-Week Online Interactive Course.

Learn more at danielfasttohealthyliving.com.

Sersie Blue & Gigi Carter

ISBN (paperback): 978-1735552910

Published by Rabbit Food Publishing

Book Cover by Hannah Lipking

To learn more about the authors and the Daniel Fast: A Bridge to Healthy Living™ program, please visit: https://danielfasttohealthyliving.com.

Follow on Instagram @danielfasttohealthyliving.

Join the Facebook Group: www.facebook.com/groups/danielfasttohealthyliving

*We are praying for you and we believe
God is going to do amazing things
during this 4-week fast.*

"Please test your servants for ten days: Give us nothing but vegetables to eat and water to drink." **Daniel 1: 12**

"In those days I, Daniel, was mourning three full weeks. I ate no pleasant food, no meat or wine came into my mouth, nor did I anoint myself at all, till three whole weeks were fulfilled." **Daniel 10: 2-3**

What are people saying about the Daniel Fast: A Bridge to Healthy Living program?

"As someone who has been through such disasters as Hurricane Katrina and now to experience the repercussions of this COVID-19 pandemic, I can tell you that it is very important for each one of us to maintain our health. When you experience a disaster, it forces you into a survivor mode. During that time period, you strive to take care of everyone else, and you tend to neglect yourself. For this reason, I commend Gigi & Sersie for recognizing and fulfilling a need through Daniel Fast: A Bridge to Healthy Living.

I saw that need when I joined the free 4-day Daniel Fast group challenge. Since my church does a Daniel Fast at the onset of each year, I knew this was the answer to get myself back on track. Due to the great results I had during the 4-day Daniel Fast, I decided to continue my journey through the 4-week Daniel Fast, to reset my journey of good health.

It feels great to be back to myself—mentally, spiritually, and physically. I am so thankful to God every morning when I awake with energy, ready to take on the challenges of each day. It's a wonderful feeling to be back on track to take care of self, in order to take care of others. After all, OUR BODIES ARE A TEMPLE."

– Donna Carter

"I did the 4-Day Daniel Fast Challenge and signed up for the 4-week course. Both Sersie and Gigi are very knowledgeable, relatable, and helpful. Not going to lie—it was not easy for me to give up sweets, chips, and bread, but I wanted to feel better and have a great quality of life as I age and was convinced this is a good way to do it. I'm 60 years old, I lost 15 pounds, 2 dress sizes down, gained muscle and my husband's cholesterol improved significantly. Check it out!"

– Susan Tompkins Schnell

"The Daniel Fast: A Bridge to Healthy Living has been a game-changer for me. The combination of the nutritional expertise of Gigi Carter and spiritual depth of Sersie Blue has been the missing piece for me. I describe my journey as more of a trip, because I've kept tripping over and tripping up. As a woman of faith, I always knew there was a connection between the call to do something about my health and the word of God, but couldn't quite build that bridge. When Gigi invited me to be a part of this program, it was like God had heard my cry. All the years of journal writing, all the years of pleas, all the shame and guilt, and trying to transition to a healthy mindset; I couldn't pivot from years and years of self-loathing. The Daniel Fast: A Bridge to Healthy Living was that missing link for me. The pivot for me has been changing the narrative, and I feel that with this program, God has given me the path. I now know that I'm worth it!"

– Mary Bogan

"I've been eating a vegan diet for 9 years, and what intrigued me was linking the spiritual part. I also had been eating a lot of processed faux meats and drinking 2-3 glasses of alcohol nightly. Going through the Daniel Fast: A Bridge to Healthy Living, my body felt better eating whole plant foods and abstaining from alcohol. I slept better, I had less joint pain, improved skin, more mental clarity, and even more energy. My husband did it with me and he lost 7 pounds and got off of one of his blood pressure medications and reduced his statin medication. I highly recommend this program for any vegan wanting a reset."

– Janne Swearengen

Preface

So, you've decided to pray and take charge of your health. We are ecstatic that you have joined the movement of thousands of people around the world who believe that God wants us healthy. Don't take this lightly: what you are doing is revolutionary. You are about your Father's business, because, you see, taking care of YOU is God's work. It is what God desires for all of us. *A Prayer for Your Health Journal* is best suited to be completed alongside the Daniel Fast: A Bridge to Healthy Living 4-Week Interactive Course. However, on its own it can be a starting point to explore healthy living.

A Prayer for Your Health Journal is much more than a string of prayers or a single prayer about one specific thing. It is a stance that you will take moving forward concerning your health. It is a way of life, a paradigm shift to seeing your health as God sees it, and to continually look to Him for guidance, direction, and inspiration when it comes to your health. It means incorporating prayer for your health even when you're achieving your health goals—not just during challenging times. It's also about learning more about plant-based nutrition and educating yourself so you can make healthy choices over the long term.

A Prayer for Your Health Journal invites God into your health journey — your areas of challenges, cravings, weight loss, emotional eating, chronic health management, you name it! It is seeing God and purpose in your health.

This journal is to be chewed slowly, never eaten in a rush. This is because as you meditate and process each day, the concepts become digestible and applicable to your daily life. Expect divine revelation and approach each day with an open heart and mind. The more you work through the devotions and apply the nutritional tips to your life, the more you will receive.

The soul of *A Prayer for Your Health Journal* is to ignite an unrelenting desire in you to live healthy so that you can live out your full purpose for the glory of God. It is designed to challenge, convict, and connect you to God's divine plan for your health.

The nutritional health nugget each day is meant to anchor you in the practical side of things so you can gain an understanding of the affect food has on your health as well as learn some simple ways to develop new habits that serve you. *A Prayer for Your Health Journal* is both compass and map: spiritual revelation and nutritional guidance all pointing you toward a bridge to healthy living.

So, buckle your seat belt and be prepared for God to change the trajectory of your health. This is not a sprint, but instead a 4-week journey toward a lifetime of better health. We are praying for you!

Gigi & Sersie

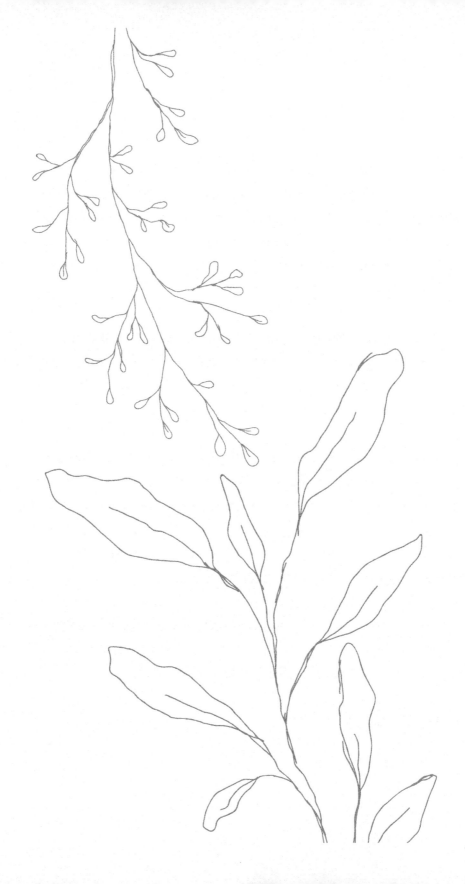

A Prayer for Your Health

I pray that God will make you whole in mind, body, and spirit.

I pray that every set goal and desire of your heart will be infused with the Holy Spirit and realized in your life in a tangible way.

I pray that you will develop new skills, draw closer to God, and break any negative relationship you have with food.

I pray that this fast will be a turning point in your health and your walk with God.

I pray that you will finish strong, energized, motivated, and renewed in spirit and body.

I pray that you will gain a deep understanding of the connection between your health and your spiritual journey.

I pray that God will break generational patterns of poor health in your family and that the cycle will end with you!

I pray that old unhealthy habits will be replaced by new habits that serve you.

I pray that you will know beyond a shadow of doubt that God wants you well! 1 Corinthians 10:31 states "so whether you eat or drink or whatever you do, do it all to the glory of God."

I pray that you will walk, talk, move your body, and eat to the glory of God!

Amen.

Sensie's Story

The Daniel Fast has a special place in my heart! It was the Daniel Fast that started my health journey. Like most Americans addicted to the standard American diet, I had an extremely poor relationship with food. During my pregnancy, my doctor diagnosed me with high blood pressure, and placed me on medications during my last trimester. Pregnant mothers with high blood pressure are at a higher risk of complications before, during, and after birth, and African American women are more likely to develop high blood pressure during pregnancy.

Birthing complications caused my son to lose oxygen to the brain, leading to illness and 24-hour care after birth. This was the most difficult season—my life hit rock bottom when he died at the age of one. I became depressed, disconnected, and desperate. Because my need to self-medicate with food was at an all-time high (oftentimes trauma creates a deeper disconnect between the body and soul), I became the heaviest I'd ever been in my life. There were also times I found myself reaching out to food to fill that void. I wasn't eating to live—I was living to eat!

As a woman of faith, I know that I need to honor God and I wanted to honor the memory of my son's life by getting healthy. That's why I was open to explore the Daniel Fast challenge offered by a friend. It was here that my road to fuller healing truly began. After completing 30 days of the fast, not only was I drawing closer to God but my blood pressure was regulated! My weight was shedding effortlessly, and my emotional health grew stronger; I was no longer depressed, and I had tons of energy. My brain fog disappeared, my mental clarity sharpened, and God's voice became clearer! Each day I woke up more energized than the day before, and was motivated to exercise.

This life-changing experience was a paradigm shift for me. After serving over a decade in ministry and working with individuals and families in the community, my focus had always been solely on emotional and spiritual wellbeing. I never connected the dots to see the influence my spirituality had on my health until now. Connecting those dots paved a new path for me in health ministries and health coaching.

Even though I'd experienced so many positive results, after the 30 days ended, I felt a sense of uncertainty. My friend had returned to her normal way of eating, so I was left with unanswered questions. I knew I wanted to maintain how I felt, but did not know where to start. I spent endless hours researching, reading, and gaining knowledge on plant-based nutrition and how it intersected with faith. One might say I was obsessed. It was during this time of education, research, and spending time with God that I realized that as a Christian I could no longer neglect my health. I knew then that God not only cares about my growth spiritually but my physical health as well! The work paid off and I navigated my way into making the Daniel Fast a way of life. It was here that The Faithful Vegan was born.

In retrospect, what I'd needed was a bridge! This is why I am so passionate about the Daniel Fast: A Bridge to Healthy Living 4-week interactive course.

This program is everything I wish I'd had and more during my experience with the Daniel Fast. My road to healing has taught me first-hand the connection between living a healthy lifestyle and exercising our faith. This experience has given me a new purpose in sharing this God-given, life-changing revelation with others so they can have the information readily available. Now I teach others how to invite God into their health journey and use their faith to affect their health. God has broadened my purpose by bringing Gigi into my life and entrusting me with the Daniel Fast: A Bridge to Healthy Living.

Gigi's Story

In 2007, as part of a routine wellness checkup, I learned that I had high cholesterol and early signs of plaque building up in my arteries. The carotid artery scan report noted that I had the arteries of a 46-year-old, yet I was only 35. My doctor wanted to put me on a statin drug. I refused, telling him I was only in my 30s and I knew what I needed to do to take better care of myself. I told him I would eat healthier foods and work out more. His response was, "Well, that's not practical and I recommend you start this medication." I politely declined and walked out.

Even without the test results, I knew I hadn't been consistent with physical activity and that my stress level was high, given the amount of traveling I did for my high-pressure job. During that period, I learned about the work of Dr. Dean Ornish and his colleagues on "The Lifestyle Heart Trial," who showed that you can reverse heart disease without the use of medications by using a whole food, plant-based diet and other lifestyle changes. Looking back on that period, I now realize that my health event was the beginning of a wakeup call that took another five years to unfold.

From ages 36 to 40, I ate what I thought was a healthy diet that included chicken breasts, cottage cheese, yogurt, skim milk, fish, eggs on weekends, and red meat about once per month. I also enjoyed vegetarian pizza loaded with cheese and veggie cheeseburgers. I was consuming between 3 and 4 servings of fruits and vegetables each day. During that period, I was following what the USDA considered to be a "healthy" dietary pattern. My cholesterol numbers improved but were still borderline. More important to me, I just didn't feel well. I was tired, sluggish, and mentally foggy. I spent an entire year going on and off "detox cleanses" to gain more energy and hopefully drop a couple pounds in the process. I even tried a cleanse that included a concoction of lemon juice, cayenne pepper, and maple syrup for five days straight. (Hey, if Beyoncé did it, it must be a good idea, right?) I felt great after fasting when I used vegetable broth and fresh juice as the transition diet, but as soon as I returned to eating my normal "healthy" diet, I quickly felt sluggish again.

In January 2012, after the holidays, I decided to transition to a vegetarian diet. I set a goal of eating vegetarian twice a week for a month, then increased it to three times a week, and so forth until the transformation was complete. I was so gung-ho about it that I put it into my development plan at work and shared it with my team. This gradual approach gave me time to figure out my go-to meals and satisfying ways to substitute vegetarian ingredients for meat. It took me six months to fully transition, but in June 2012, I at last declared "I'm a vegetarian!" I was still eating a fair amount of low-fat dairy, as well as eggs.

Only a few weeks into lacto-ovo vegetarianism, I came across two documentaries: "Forks Over Knives" and "Earthlings." After watching both, I immediately went to my husband and proclaimed I was adopting a whole food, plant-based vegan diet. Given his own health concerns, he was completely on board with joining me on this new path. It was easy once I made the decision to do it, since all I had to do at that point was remove dairy and eggs. It was by far the best decision I ever made for myself. I've had people ask me if I miss meat and dairy. Without hesitation, my response is an enthusiastic, "No!" I ate what most people eat for the first 40 years of my life, and I can say with confidence and conviction that nothing tastes as good as I feel today!

After only a few months of eating a whole food, plant-based nutrition plan, my LDL cholesterol and triglycerides dropped over 23%, and I was no longer borderline. By 2014, I was in full plant-based athletic mode, having taken up bike racing at the age of 42, and immersing myself in plant-based nutrition research. I competed and won two ultra-distance bicycle races: the RAAM 200 Florida Challenge in November 2014, and Bessie's Creek 24 in April 2015.

In 2016, after prayer and meditation, I felt called to embark on a new journey—to leave my corporate job that took me 22 years to build and go back to school to earn a Master's in Nutrition Science from the University of Alabama at Birmingham. After graduating, I launched mytrueself.com, authored and published *The Plant-Based Workplace*, and co-authored the children's book, *The Spinach in My Teeth*. More recently, I felt another calling—to partner with Sersie Blue to co-create the Daniel Fast: A Bridge to Healthy Living.

The background on how the Daniel Fast: A Bridge to Healthy Living started

God had a plan! Even though they live some 3,000 miles apart, Sersie and Gigi met during the middle of COVID-19. They shared similar but unique backgrounds in the health and wellness space. After learning that those who have a comorbidity like high blood pressure, obesity, or diabetes were dying of COVID-19 at higher rates, with a disproportionate number being from the Black community, they both knew they could not sit this one out and felt called to act. Gigi and Sersie both knew from personal and professional experience that they had the answer to prevent more needless deaths, beyond the normal practices of hand washing and wearing masks. The answer was the same thing that helped them both take control of their health: a whole food, plant-based diet and prayer!

With Gigi's nutritional background and Sersie's experience in ministry, they knew that they had just what was needed to develop a program that could change the trajectory of poor health by combining nutrition and faith. Sersie and Gigi combined their efforts with many sleepless nights and creative collaborations and developed the Daniel Fast: A Bridge to Healthy Living. Gigi and Sersie were both passionate about developing a 4-week interactive online course that would be a bridge to long-term sustainable health. They offer ongoing support via a private Facebook group with the ultimate goal to help you take control of your health and deepen your relationship with God.

Foods included and not included in the Daniel Fast: A Bridge to Healthy Living

During this fast you are expected to consume only whole plant-foods in—or close to—their most natural state. If you are a regular caffeine drinker, consider reducing your intake over two to three days before the fast starts to avoid or minimize withdrawal headaches.

Below are lists of foods included and not included in the fast.

INCLUDED	NOT INCLUDED
☑ Water	☒ All meat and animal products (poultry, beef, lamb, fish, seafood, etc.)
☑ All vegetables	
☑ All starchy vegetables (potatoes, winter squash)	☒ All dairy products (cheese, milk, cream, butter, yogurt, etc.)
☑ All fruits	☒ Eggs and related products (mayo)
☑ Mushrooms	☒ All natural and artificial sweeteners (honey, agave, sugar, stevia, molasses, maple syrup, etc.)
☑ All intact whole grains (barley, quinoa, oats, millet, amaranth, brown rice, black rice, red rice, kamut, teff)	
☑ All legumes (beans, peas, lentils)	☒ Highly processed foods (granola or energy bars, packaged frozen meals, etc.)
☑ All nuts and seeds	☒ Deep-fried foods (fries, potato chips, corn chips, etc.)
☑ Fresh herbs	

MINIMALLY PROCESSED:

☒ Leavened breads and baked goods

☑ Frozen fruit and vegetables*

☒ All oils

☑ Tofu

☒ Solid fats (margarine, lard, shortening, coconut oil, palm oil)

☑ Tempeh

☑ Corn tortilla

☒ Caffeine (coffee, tea, energy drinks)

☑ Whole wheat pasta

☒ Alcohol

☑ Canned beans*

☑ Nut butters*

☑ Carbonated water*

☑ Fresh vegetable and fruit juice*

☑ Dried herbs and seasonings

with no added sweeteners, preservatives, or artificial flavorings

IMPORTANT! PLEASE READ: The information in this program should not be used for the diagnosis or treatment of medical conditions. Always consult a doctor or other healthcare professional for diagnosis and treatment of medical conditions. If you are currently taking medication, please start by checking with your healthcare provider to determine if any adjustments need to be made to your prescription, or if this change in diet is right for you. If you use recreational drugs, consume alcohol or other controlled substances, you may experience significant withdrawal symptoms. Please contact your healthcare provider before starting this fast.

How to use this journal

This is a daily journal that coincides with the four weeks of the fast. Consider starting the fast on a Monday and having all of your preparations completed by the weekend before. Your preparations may include:

- ☐ Obtaining physician approval to do the fast.

- ☐ Clearing out your refrigerator and pantry of foods not included in the fast, that you no longer want to eat.

- ☐ Creating a simple meal plan based on the foods included in the fast.

- ☐ Completing your grocery shopping.

- ☐ Identifying a place and time of day for where and when you're going to complete the journal devotions. Be sure to carve out enough time in your schedule for quality time with God.

- ☐ Praying for God to prepare your heart to receive all the blessings He has for you during the fast.

Use the food journal to help you better understand your relationship with food. Gain insight by identifying triggers and strategies to help you be mindful and intentional about food choices.

This journal along with the dialogue and live sessions within the course is what makes the course interactive and effective.

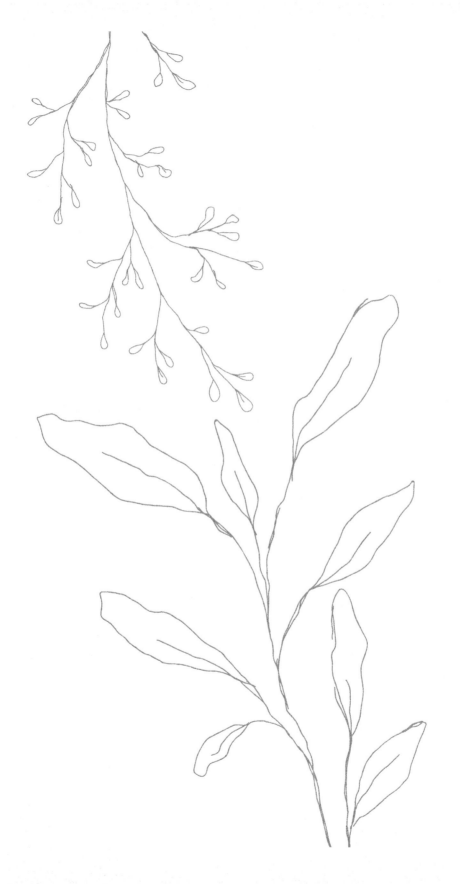

19

WEEK 1

Why our purpose is connected to our health

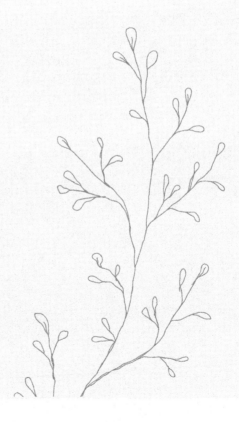

Lord help me to honor your spirit
that dwells in me,

By creating a space within my body that is
a true reflection of your glory,

Grant me the strength to walk out
my purpose in good health,

That I may not miss your perfect timing
in manifesting your will in my life

Day 1: Monday

Devotion

"God always gives us the answers to the test"

Deuteronomy 30: 19-20
Psalms 91: 9-10, 14-16

Every time we pick up our forks, we can choose life or death. The million-dollar question is: Does the food I am eating bring nourishment to my body or will it break my body down? Do not get stuck on that one bad meal or that one bad bite, because it is about what we do consistently over a period. God cares about every aspect of our lives, including what we eat.

How can you access God's strength when you are tempted?

_____

_____

How would you describe your relationship with food?

_____

_____

Health Nugget:

Drinking water throughout the day can help curb excessive eating, lower blood pressure, reduce joint pain, and improve mood and cognition. Consider working up to drinking about half of your body weight in ounces of water (or between 8-12 glasses) each day. Measure the capacity in ounces of a refillable water bottle or cup. Put one rubber band around it for each time you'll need to refill to reach your daily needs. Remove a rubber band each time you drink one full container. When all rubber bands are removed, you'll be confident knowing you hit your daily target.

Food Journal

Time	How does my body feel before eating?	What I'm eating	How does my body feel after eating?

Notes

Day 2: Tuesday

Devotion

"Stop searching outside; look within"

1 John 4: 4
Romans 8: 2, 11

God has your back! Your health matters to Him and He wants you to succeed. You have all that you need to triumph living within you. Starting a new health regimen can seem hard in the beginning, especially when you are relying on your own strength from meal to meal. Being aware of His presence during your meals and during moments of craving throughout the day will help you realize this truth. Yes! God cares that you struggle with eating that chocolate chip cookie, and He wants you to invite Him into every area of your life, big or small.

How can inviting God into every area of your life transform things?

_____

_____

_____

_____

Health Nugget:

Setting health goals can sometimes lead to establishing a specific outcome such as, "I want to lose 30 pounds" or "I want my A1C to drop to 6.5%." Instead, start with behavior-based goals that will eventually lead to weight loss and improved bloodwork, such as "Starting today, I'm going to eat 3 servings of dark leafy green vegetables daily" and "Starting tomorrow, I'm going to walk 30 minutes each day at 8:00 in the morning" This will help to keep the focus on taking action and creating healthy habits over the long term.

Food Journal

Time	How does my body feel before eating?	What I'm eating	How does my body feel after eating?

Notes

Day 3: Wednesday

Devotion

"Knowing is half the battle"

James 4: 7
Ephesians 6: 10-17

Never underestimate the enemy! When you take a step toward health, he is always lurking to distract, derail, and discourage you. Do not believe his lies. When things pop up that are challenging, dig those heels in even deeper as a declaration that you will not be stopped! Stay the course. Ramp up your prayer, draw closer to God. Keep your eyes on what is ahead.

What are the areas in your life that have the potential to distract or derail you?

_____

_____

What can you do to minimize those distractions?

_____

_____

Health Nugget:

The food groups in the Daniel Fast: A Bridge to Healthy Living program are devoid of all animal products and include vegetables, fruits, mushrooms, whole grains, legumes (e.g., beans, lentils, peas), nuts, seeds, and herbs and spices. The emphasis is on eating these foods in or close to their most natural state. Numerous studies show that eating a whole food, plant-based diet is associated with lower rates of obesity, type 2 diabetes, high cholesterol, high blood pressure and certain types of cancers. The healing power of eating whole plant foods stems from the fiber, antioxidants, and other bioactive compounds found only in these foods.

Food Journal

Time	How does my body feel before eating?	What I'm eating	How does my body feel after eating?

Notes

Day 4: Thursday

Devotion

"Food should give us life"

Genesis 1: 29
John 6: 35

God knew from the very beginning what our bodies would need to function. Food was never designed to master us; its job is to nourish us so we can thrive. With God's help we can find our way back. Fasting is a way we can redirect our hunger and thirst for food and shift it to a genuine hunger and thirst for God. Being hungry and thirsty for God is the sweet spot and where the magic happens! We become open spiritually to receive a download from God. It is the birthing ground for change.

What have you noticed about your relationship with food?

_____

_____

_____

_____

Health Nugget:

Macronutrients include carbohydrates, protein, and fat. Carbohydrates are plant-derived energy nutrients, and the primary energy source for the brain. Carbohydrates contain 4 calories per gram. Proteins are made up of amino acids and carry out critical functions in our body. Proteins contain 4 calories per gram. Fat is a necessary component of all living cells, but you only need a small amount—too much fat can lead to weight gain. Fat contains 9 calories per gram. Eating a variety of whole plant-foods, in or close to their most natural state, provides a healthy source of these macronutrients.

Food Journal

Time	How does my body feel before eating?	What I'm eating	How does my body feel after eating?

Notes

Day 5: Friday

Devotion

"Knowing the character of God is a game-changer"

Psalms 103: 1-8
Isaiah 41: 10

The only way to know God is to spend time with Him. Fasting is a gateway that facilitates intimacy with God. Do not cheat yourself: slip away any time you get to pray and mediate on His word. Pour your heart out, let Him know your struggles and your joys.

What roadblocks prevent you from opening your heart completely to God?

_____

_____

How can you be more vulnerable with God?

_____

_____

Health Nugget:

If you're trying to lose weight, calorie-density is an important concept to know. Calorie-density considers the number of calories for a given weight of food. Eating a variety of vegetables such as kale, broccoli, cauliflower, bell pepper, zucchini, celery, cucumber, collard greens, and squash, as well as fruits, mushrooms, beans, peas, lentils and intact whole grains (e.g., quinoa, brown rice, oat groats) can help you to lose weight. High calorie-density foods such as nuts and seeds should be portion-controlled, so you get some, but not too much.

Food Journal

Time	How does my body feel before eating?	What I'm eating	How does my body feel after eating?

Notes

Day 6: Saturday

Devotion

"We are co-laborers with God"

Joshua 14: 11-12
Philippians 1: 6

God wants to use us at every stage of our lives, even in our older years. Our purpose never ends. Caleb was able to actualize a promise given to him in his youth because his health was intact. Part of manifesting the dreams of our youth is having the physical, mental, and spiritual fortitude to see it through. It is so easy to place all our attention on our purpose while neglecting our health. It is only when our health fails us that we realize how important being well is to our mission. By focusing on your health, you are underwriting your purpose.

What has God called you to do in your youth that you are still working on today?

_____

_____

_____

_____

What is God calling you to do in this season and how can better health help you along that path?

Health Nugget:

One tablespoon of oil has 120 calories! One way to reduce the fat in your cooking is to use a method called dry (or water) sauté. For example, when sauteing onions, heat up a dry pan over medium heat. Add chopped raw onions to the hot pan. Oftentimes, the water from the onion will release, keeping the onions from sticking to the pan. If it doesn't, and your onions begin to stick to the pan, just add a tablespoon of water (or vegetable broth) to the hot pan and the onions will quickly release.

Food Journal

Time	How does my body feel before eating?	What I'm eating	How does my body feel after eating?

Notes

Day 7: Sunday

Devotion

"Your purpose is housed in your body"

Numbers 13
Exodus 9: 16

God can call you at any age for any purpose; it's up to you to be ready. Sometimes the dreams we had in our youth will be actualized in our later years. Do not rely solely on the strength of your youth, but live in such a way that health can follow you all the days of your life. There is no age limit for God.

How has the life of Caleb inspired you to live your best life?

_____

_____

_____

_____

_____

Health Nugget:

Part of the rationale for keeping a food journal is to help keep you focused and off "auto-pilot." Having this focus and consciousness will help you better understand your relationship with food. The Devotion on Day 4 posed the question, "What have you noticed about your relationship with food?" Now, dig deeper into to your food journal entries for the first week and answer the following questions:

1. Why do I think this?
2. Why do I believe this?
3. Who instilled this in me?
4. Where did it come from?
5. How are those thoughts and beliefs serving me, and helping me to fulfill God's purpose for me?

Food Journal

Time	How does my body feel before eating?	What I'm eating	How does my body feel after eating?

Notes

WEEK 2

Your faith is greater than your appetite

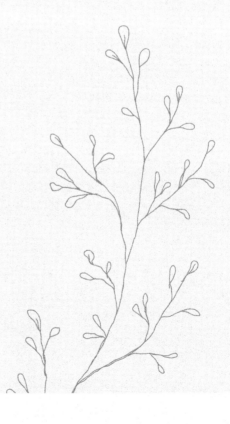

Lord grant me the wisdom to see my health as my birthright,

I pray that I will not despise the responsibility that comes with living healthfully,

I pray that I will desire the things that are a reflection of your glory,

I pray that by your grace I will have dominion over my appetite

Day 1: Monday

Devotion

Special Note: **From this day forward, take inventory and record in your journal how you feel emotionally and how connected you feel to God. Also, write down something you are grateful for each day.**

"There is always work to do when it comes to the heart"

2 Chronicles 7: 14
Romans 15: 13

Prayer and fasting always require humility. Taking this journey opens the heart up to be exposed and healed all at the same time. Putting aside our differences with others, asking for forgiveness, or letting go of our anger, fear, and resentment can open us up to hope, peace, and joy. This can dramatically affect our physical and spiritual health.

How do I feel emotionally?

_____

_____

What am I grateful for today?

_____

What does God's overflow (hope, peace, joy) look like in my life? How does that spill over into my health?

_____

_____

_____

How can prayer expose the heart and change it at the same time?

_____

_____

_____

_____

_____

Health Nugget:

Fiber is found only in whole plant-foods. Fiber plays a critical role in the health of our gut. When we eat whole plant-foods, the fiber ferments to produce short chain fatty acids. Those short chain fatty acids influence our hormones, including hunger and satiety hormones; immune system health; and our mood.

Food Journal

Time	How does my body feel before eating?	What I'm eating	How does my body feel after eating?

Notes

Day 2: Tuesday

Devotion

"Faith moves mountains"

Mark 11: 22-25
Luke 11: 34-37

Have you ever been afraid to pray about something because you did not want to be disappointed? Have you ever believed that God would not come through for you? These thoughts can be common, but don't let them stop you from praying and taking your concerns to God. Praying specifically for your health is a step of faith. Often the stress of battling a chronic illness or jumping from one diet to the other can leave us exhausted and cynical. Remember that change occurs in steps. The Daniel Fast is not a sprint or a quick fix—it is a marathon anchored in sound nutrition and faith. The journey can seem unfamiliar or even scary at times (especially in the beginning), but it helps to remember that you are on the right track!

How do I feel emotionally?

How connected to God do I feel today?

What am I grateful for today?

_____

How do I feel my life would change if I believed that God answered bold prayers?

_____

_____

How has praying for my health specifically impacted my life?

_____

_____

Health Nugget:

_____

Probiotics are the beneficial bacteria living in your gut. Prebiotics are the food for the beneficial probiotics. Prebiotics come from the fiber in whole plant-foods. Therefore, eating a diet rich in whole plant-foods allows the beneficial probiotics in our gut to thrive! Things that can deplete or harm the probiotics living in our gut include antibiotics, alcohol, poor diet, stress, poor sleep, and lack of physical activity.

_____

_____

Food Journal

Time	How does my body feel before eating?	What I'm eating	How does my body feel after eating?

Notes

Day 3: Wednesday

Devotion

"Truth"

Daniel 1
Romans 12: 1-2

Living healthfully is a spiritual practice and a compliment to God. Selah.

How do I feel emotionally?

_____

_____

_____

How connected to God do I feel today?

_____

What am I grateful for today?

_____

What does the statement above, about living healthfully, mean to me?

_____

_____

What impact does this statement have on how I view my health?

_____

_____

_____

_____

_____

_____

Health Nugget:

Eating a variety of whole plant foods provides an abundance of vitamins and minerals. Consider combining iron-rich plant-foods (such as lentils, chickpeas, beans, chia seeds, and pumpkin seeds), with vitamin C-rich foods (such as kiwi, bell pepper, broccoli, citrus fruits and tropical fruits like pineapple, guava, and papaya), because vitamin C enhances the absorption of iron.

61

Food Journal

Time	How does my body feel before eating?	What I'm eating	How does my body feel after eating?

Notes

Day 4: Thursday

Devotion

"You are enough"

Psalms 48: 9-10
Psalms 103: 1-8, 11-13

When we see God in His perfect light and we understand His loving characteristics, we can then look at ourselves correctly. It is then that we can honor and cherish every aspect of our being. God lives in us! Taking care of ourselves emotionally, physically, and spiritually demonstrates how we honor Him.

How do I feel emotionally?

_____

_____

How connected to God do I feel today?

_____

What am I grateful for today?

_____

What changes can I make in my life to ensure that I am taking care of myself physically, emotionally, and spiritually?

_____

_____

_____

_____

_____

_____

Health Nugget:

Eating a potassium-rich diet is associated with lower rates of hypertension (or high blood pressure). Potassium is also important for fluid balance, muscle contraction, and transmission of nerve impulses. A whole food, plant-based diet is rich in this important mineral, found in such foods as potatoes, berries, beans, kale, bananas, melons, flaxseeds, hemp hearts, tomatoes, and tofu.

_____

Food Journal

Time	How does my body feel before eating?	What I'm eating	How does my body feel after eating?

Notes

Day 5: Friday

Devotion

"Lean on Me"

1 John 1: 9
James 5: 16

Sometimes the hardest thing to do is let others into our areas of weakness or failure. It's easy to rely on our own strength in the hope of avoiding vulnerability. The truth is that we need each other. God designed us this way. Choosing wisely whom you let into those spaces is prudent. Accountability and fellowship are so important on this journey. Reach out, speak up, engage.

How do I feel emotionally?

_____

_____

How connected to God do I feel today?

_____

What am I grateful for today?

_____

Who can I reach out to this week for support on my wellness journey? Support may show up in a prayer or checking in with someone.

_____

_____

How do I allow God into my areas of weakness, failure, and frailty?

_____

_____

_____

_____

_____

_____

Health Nugget:

While human bodies can make vitamin D with sunlight and skin temperature, most people are deficient in this micronutrient. Geographic location, age, skin pigmentation, and use of sunscreen can make it hard to synthesize enough vitamin D from the sun. Wild mushrooms grown in ultraviolet light, and fortified foods such as orange juice with vitamin D added are the main sources of this micronutrient in a plant-based nutrition plan. Consider asking your healthcare provider about supplementing with 1,000-2,000 IU per day.

Food Journal

Time	How does my body feel before eating?	What I'm eating	How does my body feel after eating?

Notes

Day 6: Saturday

Devotion

"It is always wise to count the cost"

Genesis 25: 24-34
Hebrews 12: 16-17

Good health is our birthright. No matter what action we take, there is always a cost. Many times, we neglect this principle when it comes to what we eat or how we live out our lives concerning our health. The good news is that once we believe the truth about who God has called us to be, we no longer run from our fears—we embrace them. Taking responsibility for your health is work, but the burden is light when grounded in faith.

How do I feel emotionally?

How connected to God do I feel today?

What am I grateful for today?

What lies have I convinced myself of when it comes to taking charge of my health?

_____

How can I use God's word to counteract that?

_____

_____

What would taking responsibility for my health look like for me?

_____

_____

_____

_____

_____

Health Nugget:

Antioxidants and phytochemicals are beneficial to our health and in abundance in a whole food, plant-based dietary pattern. Eat a rainbow of fresh vegetables and fruits, as well as mushrooms, fresh herbs, intact whole grains, legumes, and some nuts and seeds daily to get the benefits of these immunity-boosting, disease-fighting foods.

Food Journal

Time	How does my body feel before eating?	What I'm eating	How does my body feel after eating?

Notes

Day 7: Sunday

Devotion

"Hungry for God"

Mathew 5: 6
Psalm 143: 6

Fasting and prayer is a beautiful way to master our physical appetites and deepen our hunger for God. The more we tap into our hunger for God, the more we can access His strength to overcome our physical appetites. All our deepest needs can be met only on a soul level as we hunger for God.

How do I feel emotionally?

_____

How connected to God do I feel today?

_____

What am I grateful for today?

_____

What would waiting on God during uncomfortable moments of temptation look like for me?

_____

How will meditating on God's word help me in those moments?

_____

_____

How has God shown up for me so far during this fast?

_____

_____

_____

_____

_____

Health Nugget:

Omega 3 alpha-linolenic acid (ALA), an essential fatty acid, is associated with improved heart and brain health. Omega 3 ALA is found in chia seeds, flaxseeds (ground flax is preferred for better absorption), hemp hearts, and walnuts. Adding 1 to 2 tablespoons to your salad, smoothie, or oatmeal each day can help you get the recommended dietary allowance of this important nutrient. Be sure to mix it up. Choose chia seeds to add to your smoothie one day, and ground flaxseeds the next day. Alternatively, add 1 tablespoon of chia seeds plus 1 tablespoon of chopped walnuts to your overnight oats. Remember, variety is key!

Food Journal

Time	How does my body feel before eating?	What I'm eating	How does my body feel after eating?

Notes

WEEK 3

Meeting our needs with God, not food

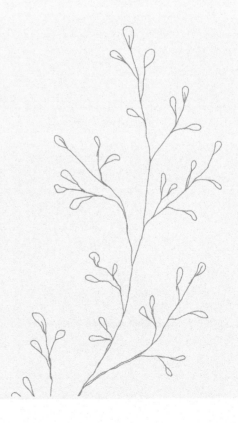

I pray that I will understand
the truth behind my thirst,

Help me to find rest, peace,
purpose, and joy in you,

Tear down any idols that I
have created in my life,

So that I may be completely
free to walk in your light

Day 1: Monday

Devotion

"Man cannot live by bread alone"

Luke 11: 2-4
Mathew 4: 4

Isn't it funny how food can consume our lives if we are not careful? Have you ever found yourself eating a meal and at the same time preparing in your mind what you will eat next? Our obsession with food can cloud our judgment. That's why doing this fast and breaking our emotional dependence on food is an act of worship. It is pushing back against our physical desires in order to elevate our spiritual awareness and connection to God.

How do I feel emotionally?

_____

_____

How connected to God do I feel today?

_____

What am I grateful for today?

_____

How has the Daniel Fast helped me gain spiritual awareness?

_____

_____

What have I noticed about my thoughts around food during the Daniel Fast?

_____

_____

_____

_____

Health Nugget:

Combine leafy greens with avocado (or another healthy plant fat) for as much as 7x lutein absorption. Lutein is part of the carotenoid family of phytochemicals and is known for its anti-inflammatory properties and benefits for eye health.

Food Journal

Time	How does my body feel before eating?	What I'm eating	How does my body feel after eating?

Notes

Day 2: Tuesday

Devotion

"God's word is a light"

Joshua 1: 8-9
Psalms 23: 1-4, 6

There is power in meditating on God's word until it sinks into the crevices of our souls. Repetition is the mother of skill; you cannot manifest the promises of God in your life unless you merge what is on the pages to your heart. Reading, singing, mediating, studying, repeating, speaking aloud, and memorizing are some of the ways you can illuminate the word of God into your life.

How do I feel emotionally?

_____

_____

How connected to God do I feel today?

_____

What am I grateful for today?

_____

How can I make more time to meditate on God's word?

_____

_____

How can I get creative with the way I meditate on God's word?

_____

_____

_____

_____

Health Nugget:

Combine room-temperature tomatoes with avocado or other healthy plant fat to enhance absorption of lycopene. Lycopene is also a part of the carotenoid family and known to be beneficial for heart health and protective against cancer.

Food Journal

Time	How does my body feel before eating?	What I'm eating	How does my body feel after eating?

Notes

Day 3: Wednesday

Devotion

"There is a season for everything"

Ecclesiastes 3: 1-8
Matthew 5: 4

Have you ever considered that you are right where God wants you to be? Do you believe that today is your season to take hold of your health? God has led you to this point in life for a reason. The road has not been easy, but you have not given up. Change sometimes causes us to mourn the old even as we embrace the new. But God sees us just where we are. He comforts us through it all.

How do I feel emotionally?

_____

_____

How connected to God do I feel today?

_____

What am I grateful for today?

_____

What is God trying to teach me in this season of my life?

_____

_____

What is usually my natural response to change?

_____

_____

_____

Health Nugget:

Eat turmeric-containing dishes, such as yellow curry, with a small sprinkle of black pepper and a small amount of healthy plant fats. This combination helps to improve the absorption of curcuminoids through the lymphatics, which is part of your immune system. Curcumin is known for its anti-inflammatory properties.

Food Journal

Time	How does my body feel before eating?	What I'm eating	How does my body feel after eating?

Notes

Day 4: Thursday

Devotion

"God knows what we need more than we do"

Ephesians 3: 20
2 Corinthians 9: 8

God always gives us what need and more than we anticipated. However, He does not always show up exactly the way we penciled it out for Him. Do you remember as a child, when you were still learning to write, that you were always being told not to write in pen to allow for correction? As children of God we should not pray in "pen" because we need to leave room for correction. Praying in pencil allows you to accept that your plans are not always the best way; thus, you can erase your desires from your heart and accept God's perfect will for your life.

How do I feel emotionally?

_____

_____

How connected to God do I feel today?

_____

What am I grateful for today?

_____

What desires have I written in "pen" on my heart?

_____

_____

What roadblocks are preventing me from trusting God completely?

_____

_____

_____

_____

_____

Health Nugget:

Leave watermelon on the kitchen counter. When it's not exposed to cold, watermelon has 40% more lycopene and 139% more beta-carotene than watermelon stored in the refrigerator, according to one study.

Food Journal

Time	How does my body feel before eating?	What I'm eating	How does my body feel after eating?

Notes

Day 5: Friday

Devotion

"Your health is a gift"

James 1: 17
1 Chronicles 16: 11-12

By now it's established that God wants you healthy, but how that journey will unfold will be unique to you. We are each only given one life on earth, one body. Living in a way that honors that concept opens you up to demonstrate love, grace, and compassion to yourself and those around you. Reframing your life as a gift awakens your spiritual antennas to receive and distribute gratitude.

How do I feel emotionally?

_____

_____

How connected to God do I feel today?

_____

What am I grateful for today?

How does reframing my life and body as a gift influence the way I approach my health?

How can my life well-lived be a gift to others?

Health Nugget:

Lean towards eating more local and seasonal. When food is picked fresh out of your own garden or is from a local farmer it not only tastes better, but it's more nutritious than eating produce that's been shipped from thousands of miles away and sitting on store shelves for days (possibly weeks) before consumption. Of course, if supermarket produce is the only choice, go for it. But when given the option of local, go for that!

Food Journal

Time	How does my body feel before eating?	What I'm eating	How does my body feel after eating?

Notes

Day 6: Saturday

Devotion

"Food for the soul"

John 4: 1-26
Psalm 143: 6

Quenching one's physical thirst with water is innate to the human experience. Trying to quench an emotional or spiritual thirst with the same water is counterproductive. All emotional and spiritual emptiness can only be filled from a spiritual source.

How do I feel emotionally?

_____

_____

_____

How connected to God do I feel today?

_____

What am I grateful for today?

_____

What are my top three triggers when it comes to emotional eating?

_____

_____

What key indicators can I use to identify when I am experiencing physical hunger versus an emotional/spiritual hunger?

_____

_____

_____

_____

_____

Health Nugget:

Add 2 teaspoons of vinegar to high carbohydrate meals such as whole grain pastas, potatoes, and rice dishes. One study showed that adding vinegar will reduce the spike in blood sugar, insulin, and triglycerides by approximately 20% within the same hour.

Food Journal

Time	How does my body feel before eating?	What I'm eating	How does my body feel after eating?

Notes

Day 7: Sunday

Devotion

"Heal your heart, find your purpose"

John 14: 1
Mathew 11: 28

Many times, our purpose is hidden behind a broken heart, and this is where we can lose sight of our dreams. Once we begin to heal, our purpose shines bright again. Broken hearts are our road miles from living. No one is exempt. Giving our hearts a tune-up through prayer and fasting is the reset we all need.

How do I feel emotionally?

_____

_____

How connected to God do I feel today?

_____

What am I grateful for today?

_____

What new or renewed insights around purpose has God revealed to me during this fast?

_____

_____

What new behavior will I replace with the next time I am tempted to use food to solve a problem and/or stressor in my life?

_____

_____

_____

_____

Health Nugget:

Meal planning can help set you up for success. Taking some time to plan out your meals will take the guesswork out of what you're going to eat throughout the week. Consider meal prepping twice a week (e.g., Sundays and Wednesdays) to batch-cook staples such as beans, rice, and steel cut oats. Also, organize and freeze fruits (e.g., berries, mango, grapes), veggies (e.g., tomatoes, kale, spinach) to be used in smoothies, sauces, and soups. Finally, have some "go-to" meals in the freezer you can pull out and warm up (e.g., veggie burgers, soups, veggie burritos).

Food Journal

Time	How does my body feel before eating?	What I'm eating	How does my body feel after eating?

Notes

WEEK 4

The power of saying grace

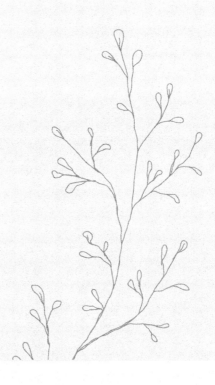

Lord help me to stir up the
gift of gratitude in my life,

I pray that I will acknowledge
you in my everyday living,

I pray that I will eat in the
best interest of my health,

I pray that my values will
align with my plate

Day 1: Monday

Devotion

"Grace is enough"

1 Corinthians 10: 13
2 Corinthians 12: 8-10

Have you ever prayed that God would remove your desire for certain foods? Even though you are beginning to enjoy your new way of eating, consider those stressful times when you find yourself craving those chocolate chip cookies. Now that you have started eating primarily whole foods, the cravings you've experienced in the past greatly decrease. But living healthy does not mean you never crave certain foods; it just means you have the strength to pass them up. Tapping into God's grace during these moments is what builds us up and deepens our relationship with God.

How do I feel emotionally?

How connected to God do I feel today?

What am I grateful for today?

_____

How does knowing that God's grace is enough help me when I face temptations?

_____

_____

What is different in how I handle my cravings now versus before I started the fast?

_____

_____

_____

_____

_____

Health Nugget:

Vitamin B12 is made from bacteria found in the soil and in water streams. The main sources of this micronutrient in a plant-based diet are fortified foods such as nutritional yeast, plant-based milks, and cereals. Check with your healthcare provider about whether supplementation of vitamin B12 is right for you.

Food Journal

Time	How does my body feel before eating?	What I'm eating	How does my body feel after eating?

Notes

Day 2: Tuesday

Devotion

"New beginnings are the best start"

2 Corinthians 5: 17
Colossians 3: 9-11

By now you may have developed a new way of thinking about your health. Perhaps you count several ways eating whole foods combined with praying has benefited you. Seeing this fast as a new beginning will empower you to continue beyond the fast. New beginnings are always the best way to start, because they assume that we are leaving the unwanted habits in the past. You are at a crossroads with your health, and seeing this moment as a new beginning will shape how you move forward.

How do I feel emotionally?

How connected to God do I feel today?

116

What am I grateful for today?

Will this fast end or be a bridge to healthy living?

How does seeing this fast as a new beginning push me to turn my new habits into a lifestyle?

Health Nugget:

Iodine is a mineral involved in thyroid hormone regulation. Too much or too little of it can cause thyroid issues like hypothyroidism and goiter. Iodine deficiency was a public health issue in many countries, including the United States in the early 1900s. After salt producers started adding iodine to table salt, the concern subsided. The main sources of iodine in a plant-based diet are sea vegetables (e.g., nori seaweed, wakame) and iodized salt. Check with your healthcare provider about whether supplementation of iodine is right for you.

Food Journal

Time	How does my body feel before eating?	What I'm eating	How does my body feel after eating?

Notes

Day 3: Wednesday

Devotion

"A new thing"

Isaiah 43: 18-19
2 Corinthians 4: 16-17

Are you still traumatized from all those times you starved yourself, or decided to complete a crash diet with a friend at work only to find yourself right back where you started? Are you skeptical that eating "real" whole foods is the answer to your health dilemma? The difference here is that you invited God into this space. This new understanding of the connection between our faith and our health may seem different, complex, and radical all at the same time. However, it is actually intuitively simple; the complexity comes when we try satisfying our own desires. God wants you healthy, He always has. He was just waiting for you to buy into it. God is doing a new thing concerning your health!

How do I feel emotionally?

How connected to God do I feel today?

What am I grateful for today?

_____

How strongly do I believe that God wants me healthy? And how does that belief shape how I will move forward after the fast is over?

_____

_____

_____

In what ways do I feel God is doing a new thing concerning my health?

_____

_____

_____

_____

Health Nugget:

If you like how you're feeling eating a whole food, plant-based diet, consider making it your new normal.

_____

_____

Food Journal

Time	How does my body feel before eating?	What I'm eating	How does my body feel after eating?

Notes

Day 4: Thursday

Devotion

"A prayer for your health"

1 Thessalonians 5: 16-18
Ephesians 6: 18

Never stop praying for your health! Prayer without ceasing keeps you close to God and keeps your health goals at the forefront. A prayer for your health is not one prayer, or a 4-week Daniel Fast. It's living out a healthy life with God in the center of it. The very act of denying yourself toxic foods and meditating on God's word is a prayer for your health. Getting rid of negative mindsets and moving your body is a prayer for your health. Deciding to only put healthy foods into your body is a prayer for your health. Being kind to yourself is a prayer for your health. Knowing your triggers is a prayer for your health. Tapping into the power of the Holy Spirit to walk in health is a prayer for your health. You see, a prayer for your health is the constant balancing act of living out our lives for God's glory.

How do I feel emotionally?

How connected to God do I feel today?

What am I grateful for today?

_____

How can I make praying for my health a lifestyle?

_____

_____

In what ways can I improve my prayer life?

_____

_____

_____

_____

_____

Health Nugget:

If you're planning to make a whole food, plant-based nutrition plan your new normal, figure out your 8-10 go-to meals and 3-5 go-to snacks that are easy to prepare and enjoyable. Having this thought through will reduce any stress you may have about what you're going to eat.

Food Journal

Time	How does my body feel before eating?	What I'm eating	How does my body feel after eating?

Notes

Day 5: Friday

Devotion

"Gratitude changes our actions"

Psalm 9: 1
Daniel 2: 23

The awesome thing about gratitude is that it changes us. It changes the way we view the world and it alters our actions. It is impossible to remain stuck, defeated, or complacent with a grateful heart. Sustaining the changes you've made starts with gratitude. Count your wins and see your failures as a teacher during this health journey. Gratitude will uproot habits that do not serve you and open your heart to the leading of the Holy Spirit.

How do I feel emotionally?

How connected to God do I feel today?

What am I grateful for today?

_____

How has documenting what I am grateful for each day impacted my life?

_____

_____

How can I practice more gratitude in my life?

_____

_____

_____

_____

_____

Health Nugget:

Using your food journal, identify key strategies that you'll use to deal with triggers. For example, if you know that stressful conversations with coworkers or family can lead to over-eating junk food, know that it's a trigger and then figure out your strategy, such as to take a walk or to find a quiet room to close your eyes and focus on your breath, or to grab a bag of celery sticks to eat instead.

Food Journal

Time	How does my body feel before eating?	What I'm eating	How does my body feel after eating?

Notes

Day 6: Saturday

Devotion

"The Power of Saying Grace"

Genesis 1: 26-29
Ephesians 5: 2

Eating has become a familiar part of our daily routine — most days we eat without thinking about it. We are bombarded by food; it is everywhere and at our fingertips. Because we have become so familiar with food, we underestimate the power it has to heal us. Thus, we are also disconnected from how much food can harm us. We are living on auto-pilot, often eating out of alignment with our best interests. Saying grace from the perspective of "does this food honor my body and God" is our way back home. When we slow down, breathe, assess, and pause as we say grace, it then can shock us out of auto-pilot to engage with our plate again.

How do I feel emotionally?

How connected to God do I feel today?

What am I grateful for today?

_____

In what ways can you redefine how you say grace?

_____

_____

_____

_____

_____

_____

_____

Health Nugget:

Some strategies for handling social functions and family gatherings may include: eating before you go, having a go-to snack handy, taking a healthy plant-based entrée to share with others, and shifting the focus of the gathering from food to an activity.

Food Journal

Time	How does my body feel before eating?	What I'm eating	How does my body feel after eating?

Notes

Day 7: Sunday

Devotion

"Food is political"

1 Timothy 1: 5
1 Corinthians 16: 14

How does food get to your table and under what conditions? Explore this question. Deciding on how much ownership you take in answering this question is a spiritual journey in and of itself. Pull on the attributes of God to guide you: love, kindness, mercy, honor, peace, and grace.

How do I feel emotionally?

How connected to God do I feel today?

What am I grateful for today?

_____

What impact does a "conscious" understanding of saying grace have in your life?

_____

_____

How do love and empathy shape the way you view what you eat?

_____

_____

_____

_____

Health Nugget:

Eating whole food, plant-based leaves a lighter environmental footprint and reduces the suffering of animals. Your personal health is supported when the planet is sustained with healthy agriculture, and you're living out your ethical values of kindness and love towards those with whom you share this earth.

Food Journal

Time	How does my body feel before eating?	What I'm eating	How does my body feel after eating?

Notes

Consider the adoption of a whole food, plant-based dietary pattern as your new normal. While the 4-week fast includes much of what you'd eat on a "normal" and healthful diet, there are some foods you can consider introducing provided none of these are considered "trigger" foods that result in over-indulging and over-eating.

Foods you may want to add include:

Whole grain breads. Our favorite supermarket brand is Ezekiel, Food for Life, but there are others. Just read the label to ensure there aren't added preservatives or animal products. Or consider making your own! Whole grain breads are a great way to enjoy avocado toast and peanut butter and banana sandwiches.

Natural sweeteners, such as maple syrup and agave. While you'll want to be careful with the quantities used, since they are very calorie-dense, these sweeteners can help balance out flavors when used in small amounts in spicy dishes such as curry or chili. They are also helpful in balancing out taste if you've added vinegar to your grains.

Commercially produced plant-based milks. While homemade plant-milks are delicious, commercially prepared can be convenient and a time saver. These milks may also be a good source of fortified vitamins and minerals, such as vitamin B12, calcium, and vitamin D. Be sure to read the labels and choose plant-based milks that don't have added sugar or oils.

Oils. In most cases, refined oils are not necessarily "healthy" when compared to the whole foods where those oils originated, but small amounts of can be added back into an overall healthful whole food, plant-based nutrition plan. Arguably, the healthy oils include flaxseed oil (use in cold dishes or smoothies only), extra virgin olive oil, walnut oil, sesame oil, and avocado oil. Avoid coconut oil and palm oil due to the high levels of saturated fat. If weight loss is a concern, it may be best to avoid all oil due to its high calorie-density of 120 calories per tablespoon.

Dark chocolate. The cocoa in dark chocolate contains flavanols, a beneficial plant chemical shown to improve heart health. This "treat" can be added in small amounts as part of an overall healthful whole food, plant-based nutrition plan. However, due to its high calorie-density—and for some, addictive nature—it may be best to avoid. Flavanols can be consumed by eating grapes, kale, and peaches too.

Pastas. Consider avoiding white refined pastas, but expand from the whole wheat pasta to include chickpea, lentil, and other legume-based pastas.

And remember: never stop praying for your health!

Philippians 1: 6
"God is the one who began this good work in you, and I am certain that he won't stop before it is complete on the day that Christ Jesus returns."

The journey doesn't end here. It is the beginning of something great concerning your health! The seeds that you've planted over these 4 weeks—know that God is faithful to bring them to fruition.

Be kind to yourself. It's not about perfection, but instead taking steps in the direction to add more whole plant foods into your life.

For ongoing support and encouragement, please join the Facebook Group Page: *https://www.facebook.com/groups/danielfasttohealthyliving*

Made in the USA
Coppell, TX
13 August 2021